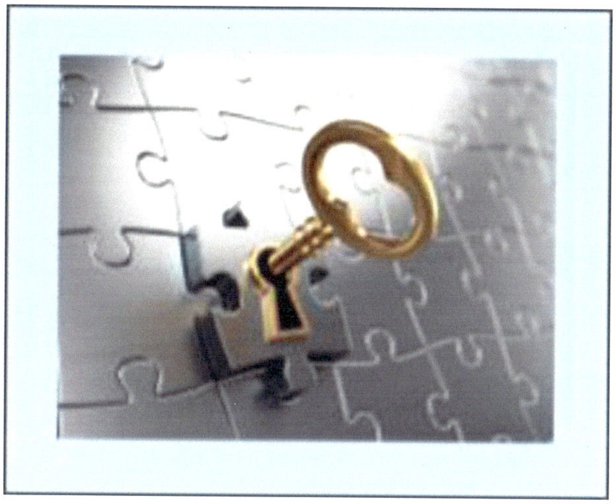

Keys to Success

How to Study for NCLEX-RN®
and Feel Ready to Practice

Lori A. Ballard MSN, RN

Copyrights

The teaching methods and opinions expressed are solely that of the author which is protected under academic freedom and does not belong to the university of which I am employed. The original work of nursing theorists Ida Jean Orlando and psychology's Abraham H. Maslow, NCSBN's NCLEX-RN Test Plan® and NANDA® International Nursing Diagnoses Definitions and Classifications 2021-2023 remain intact. Information within each has been compared, matched and cross-referenced.

About the Author

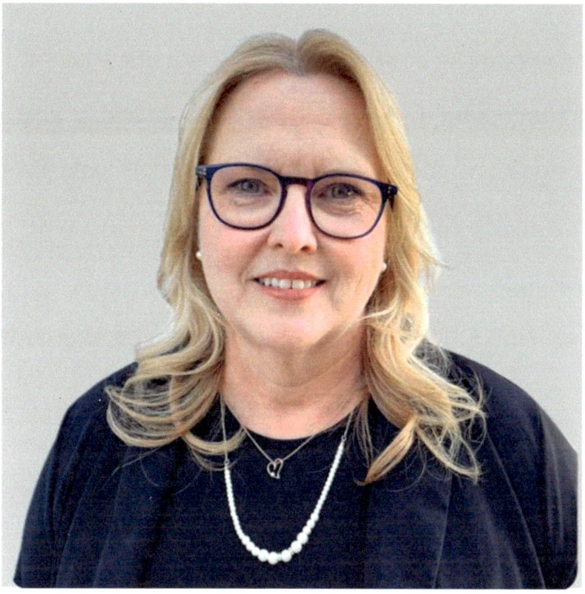

Lori A. Ballard MSN, RN

I have been a BSN Registered Nurse since 1989. I have ten years of perioperative nursing (circulating, post-anesthesia care, same day surgery and endoscopy), three years of gastroenterology, office endoscopy and office management, a few years of home health and hospital administrative case management. In 2001 I returned to bedside nursing. I worked in a float pool briefly, then transferred to the emergency department, urgent care, triage and was a relief supervisor for approximately three years. In 2004 returned to the previous gastroenterology physician's office briefly then began working at my alma mater's student health clinic in 2006. It was there I completed my master's degree in nurse education. I started teaching in our BSN program in 2011. I have been helping students prepare for NCLEX-RN® since 2015. My personal experiences as a struggling student, years of bedside nursing, and assisting hundreds of graduating seniors puts me in a unique position to help you too.

Dedication

This book is dedicated to the nursing students and new nurses who want to do more than the bare minimum it takes to pass an exam or make it through another shift. The information I have reorganized will help you think about things differently which can make a huge difference in how well you understand and critically think. In this book I will share with you how to efficiently sort through what you have already learned in order to demonstrate your clinical judgment in the classroom, during your licensure exam and most importantly, while caring for the populations you serve.

Disclaimer

This book should be used to supplement with the licensure preparation resources you already have. The original work of nursing theorists Ida Jean Orlando and philosophy's Abraham H. Maslow, NCSBN's NCLEX-RN Test Plan® and NANDA International Nursing Diagnoses Definitions and Classifications 2021-2023® remain intact. *Information within each has been compared, matched together, and cross-referenced. You won't find all this all-in-one source anywhere else to date.* The Keys to Success will review essential resources to use. It also provides suggestions on a systematic way to study. This book is not emphasizing formal NANDA International® language or the process of writing a care plan by those standards. For the sake of time and avoiding redundancy *this book does not include complete care plans or comprehensive details of the NCLEX-RN® test plan. You will need to review those original sources.*

Table Of Contents

Caring & Connecting the Dots

Figuring out how to study for NCLEX is overwhelming and rightfully so. You have resources from class work, textbooks, online products, and endless apps. I've seen a lot of students try to use too many products at once, only to find out they hadn't used their time and resources well at all. I'm going to give you a prioritized way to study that will prepare you for the eighty-five-question licensure exam. Don't think about this process as over-preparing. What you are really doing is preparing for practice.

Having your license and still not knowing what to do is terrifying. Key to preparation is to study standardized care plans. A care plan book contains everything we are supposed to teach you to do as a nurse. These are all things you are expected to do without being told. Meaning, you won't have an order to prompt you. Yet, these interventions are essential to safe patient care *and* you are expected to initiate their actions. They are the standard of practice for a generalized nurse. *How else are you supposed to figure out what to do, when you don't know what you are doing yet?*

I realize many students and faculty alike, view care plans as an outdated clinical assignment or an insignificant part of the patient's admission process. The advice in this book is a bit of a work-around. You may feel like you are studying backwards. But, trust me when I say, studying standardized care plans will definitely help you bridge gaps, recognize patterns, and understand better, so you don't have to memorize so much.

A Quick Story About How I Know This Will Work

As an educator I have always felt strongly about the importance of the nursing process and care plans. This has much to do with the vivid memory of my NCLEX-RN® exam. I was not a good test taker at all. I struggled with test anxiety and read at a very slow pace. I remember crying myself to sleep the night before my NCLEX-RN®. During my exam, I was able to calm myself because the realization hit me that the questions were essentially care plans. Luckily for me, I had done care plans on most of the client scenarios I was tested over. I gained even more respect for care planning during my time as a case manager. I learned so much about how hospitals function as a whole. Care plans aren't just another piece of admission paperwork or screen to click through. Regulatory bodies enforce strict fines when care plans are not initiated and updated timely. Case management taught me that my job was managing the care plan from admission to discharge. Care plans became most important to me during my transitions into new specialties. Going from highly specialized nursing and administrative responsibilities back to bedside nursing was not easy. I felt like a brand-new nurse every time and essentially, I was. Having a good understanding of common care plans helped me prioritize the care I gave while I was still learning practice standards unique to that specialty. I know this will work because it worked for me. I've also seen countless students use this process to catch up and improve their test scores in just a matter of weeks. This mentoring process has inspired me to share what **I am most passionate about…Your Success!**

The Why behind the What

Care plans are nothing new. As early as the 1930s nurses used care plans to instruct less educated assistants on tasks that needed to be completed for their patients (Dellefieldp.128). In fact, the care plan format that I used during nursing school referred to nursing interventions as "nursing orders". The defined nursing process as we know it today is relatively new. Ida Jean Orlando published The Dynamic Nurse-Patient Relationship in 1961. Her theory maintains the nursing process relies on human interactions to create the nurse-patient relationship. Care plans didn't start using formal language and a unified process until after the formation of The North American Nursing Diagnosis (NANDA) International in 1973. They standardized the current terminology, define the process of care planning, approve and classify nursing diagnoses. There are currently thirteen domains and two hundred and forty-nine recognized nursing diagnoses (NANDA International p. 109).

Orlando also encompassed Maslow's Hierarchy of Needs into the Nursing Process (Orlando 1961). As I'm sure you already know, A.H. Maslow is the psychologist whose theory states human needs must be met in a prioritized manner before advancing to the next higher tier. The five categories advance from basic to self-fulfillment needs (Maslow 1943).

Because the Nursing Process incorporates Malsow's Hierarchy of Needs, and the NCLEX-RN® test plan integrates the Nursing Process into every question (RN Test Plan, April 2023), using the hierarchy of needs to help answer priority questions is often recommended as a test taking technique.

Very simply defined, care plans are symptoms &/or risk management. You don't have to wait until all the course work in your curriculum is complete to start applying the essentials of nursing.

Having a good foundational understanding of the nursing process, approved diagnosis, prioritized goals and corresponding nursing interventions will give you the extra resources you need. Exams ask you, "what are you going to do?". Care plan books are the only resource you have that tell you nothing but what to do. It's also a very efficient way to study, especially when you don't have time to do content specific work. All you need is a good care plan book and the list of nursing diagnoses in this book. I recommend a pocket size desk copy that prioritizes nursing goals then lists specific nursing interventions that correspond to each goal. Remember you are studying standardized care plans. Some interventions listed in your care plan book may not apply to every scenario.

The most important why to do the extra work is ***because you care!*** You aren't just studying the bare minimum required just to pass exams. Understanding care plans and recognizing when to use their interventions will build confidence, strengthen your critical thinking skills and give you the resources you need to provide safe and competent care.

EXACTLY WHAT TO DO

Specifically, I want you to study standardized care plans that are organized by Maslow's Hierarchy of Needs. I have used Maslow's original three main categories to help with pattern recognition. First is Basic Needs which includes physiological and safety needs. Second is Psychological Needs of belongingness, love and esteem needs. And third is Self-fulfillment Needs, Self-Actualization. Because most care plan books will also categorize diagnosis by NANDA-I Nursing Domains®, I will list the domains, then list the corresponding nursing diagnoses in no particular order. You will then need to use your care plan book to look up the diagnosis definition, risk factors, at risk population, associated conditions, goals and interventions. I have the nursing diagnoses bulleted so you can use this section as a checklist. Skim through everything first. Check off the ones you already know, then focus on reviewing the remaining diagnoses. Chances are good you are very familiar with many care plans on this list.

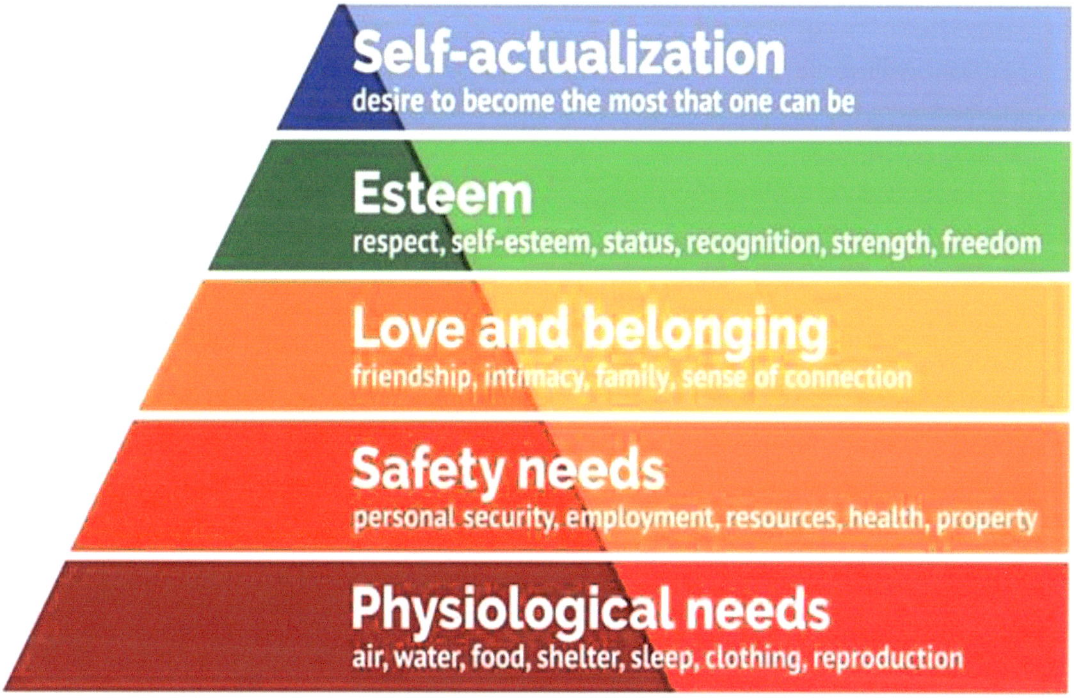

Maslow's hierarchy of needs

Nursing Diagnoses Listed by Maslow's Hierarchy of Needs

Basic Needs

Physiological Needs

Physiological needs are things necessary for human survival. This includes air, food, during shelter, clothing, warmth, sex, and sleep. The corresponding NANDA-I Nursing Domains® include Nutrition, Elimination and Exchange, Activity and Rest, Perception and Cognition, Sexuality, Growth and Development.

- Imbalanced nutrition: less than body requirements
- Readiness for enhanced nutrition
- Insufficient breast milk production
- Ineffective breastfeeding
- Interrupted breastfeeding
- Readiness for enhanced breastfeeding
- Ineffective adolescent eating dynamics
- Ineffective child eating dynamics
- Ineffective infant feeding dynamics
- Obesity
- Overweight
- Risk for overweight
- Ineffective infant suck-swallow response
- Impaired swallowing
- Risk for unstable blood glucose
- level
- Neonatal hyperbilirubinemia
- Risk for neonatal hyperbilirubinemia
- Risk for impaired liver function
- Risk for metabolic syndrome
- Risk for electrolyte imbalance
- Risk for imbalanced fluid volume
- Deficient fluid volume
- Risk for deficient fluid volume
- Excess fluid volume (Herdman, Kamitsuru, Lopes p. 211-212).
- Disability-associated urinary incontinence
- Impaired urinary elimination
- Mixed urinary incontinence
- Stress urinary incontinence
- Urge urinary incontinence
- Risk for urge urinary incontinence
- Urinary retention
- Risk for urinary retention
- Constipation
- Risk for constipation
- Perceived constipation
- Chronic functional constipation
- Risk for chronic functional constipation mobility
- Impaired bowel continence
- Diarrhea

BASIC NEEDS

- Dysfunctional gastrointestinal motility
- Risk for dysfunctional gastrointestinal motility
- Impaired gas exchange (Herdman, Kamitsuru, Lopes p. 247-248).
- Insomnia
- Sleep deprivation
- Readiness for enhanced sleep
- Disturbed sleep pattern
- Decreased activity tolerance
- Risk for decreased activity tolerance
- Risk for disuse syndrome
- Impaired bed mobility
- Impaired physical mobility
- Impaired wheelchair mobility
- Impaired sitting, Impaired standing
- Impaired transfer ability
- Impaired walking
- Imbalanced energy field
- Fatigue
- Wandering
- Ineffective breathing pattern
- Decreased cardiac output
- Risk for decreased cardiac output
- Risk for impaired cardiovascular function
- Ineffective lymphedema self-management
- Risk for ineffective lymphedema self-management
- Impaired spontaneous ventilation
- Risk for unstable blood pressure
- Risk for thrombosis
- Risk for decreased cardiac tissue perfusion
- Risk for ineffective cerebral tissue perfusion
- Ineffective peripheral tissue perfusion
- Risk for ineffective peripheral tissue perfusion
- Dysfunctional ventilatory weaning response
- Dysfunctional adult ventilatory weaning response
- Bathing self-care deficit
- Dressing self-care deficit
- feeding self-deficit
- Toileting self-care deficit
- Readiness for enhanced self-care
- Self-neglect (Herdman, Kamitsuru, Lopes p. 271-273).

Safety Needs

Safety needs pertain to protection from elements, security, order, law, stability and freedom from fear. The corresponding NANDA-I Nursing Domains® include Safely and Protection Coping/Stress Tolerance, and Comfort.

- Risk for infection
- Risk for dry mouth
- Risk for surgical site infection
- Risk for adult falls
- Ineffective airway clearance
- Risk for child falls
- Risk for aspiration
- Risk for injury
- Risk for bleeding
- Risk for corneal injury
- Impaired dentition
- Nipple-areolar complex injury
- Risk for dry eye
- Risk for nipple-areolar complex
- Ineffective dry eye injury self-management
- Risk for dry mouth
- Risk for adult falls
- Risk for child falls
- Risk for injury
- Risk for corneal injury
- Nipple-areolar complex injury
- Risk for nipple-areolar complex injury
- Risk for urinary tract injury
- Risk for perioperative positioning injury
- Risk for thermal injury
- Impaired oral mucous membrane integrity
- Risk for impaired oral mucous membrane integrity
- Risk for peripheral neurovascular dysfunction
- Risk for physical trauma
- Risk for vascular trauma
- Adult pressure injury
- Risk for adult pressure injury
- Child pressure injury
- Risk for child pressure injury
- Neonatal pressure injury
- Risk for neonatal pressure injury
- Risk for shock Impaired skin integrity
- Risk for impaired skin integrity
- Risk for sudden infant death
- Risk for suffocation
- Delayed surgical recovery
- Risk for delayed surgical recovery Impaired tissue integrity
- Risk for impaired tissue integrity
- Risk for female genital mutilation
- Risk for other-directed violence
- Risk for self-directed violence
- Self-mutilation
- Risk for self-mutilation
- Risk for suicidal behavior
- Contamination
- Risk for contamination

- Risk for occupational injury
- Risk for poisoning
- Risk for adverse reaction to iodinated contrast media
- Risk for allergy reaction
- Risk for latex allergy reaction
- Hyperthermia
- Hypothermia
- Risk for hypothermia
- Neonatal hypothermia
- Risk for neonatal hypothermia
- Risk for perioperative hypothermia
- Ineffective thermoregulation
- Risk for ineffective thermoregulation (Herdman, Kamitsuru, Lopes p. 463-465).
- Risk for complicated immigration transition
- Post-trauma syndrome
- Risk for post-trauma syndrome
- Rape-trauma syndrome
- Relocation stress syndrome
- Risk for relocation stress syndrome
- Ineffective activity planning
- Risk for ineffective activity planning
- Anxiety
- Defensive coping
- Ineffective coping
- Readiness for enhanced community coping
- Compromised family coping
- Disabled family coping
- Readiness for enhanced family Coping
- Death anxiety
- Ineffective denial
- Fear
- Maladaptive Grieving
- Risk for maladaptive grieving
- Impaired mood regulation
- Powerlessness
- Risk for powerlessness
- Readiness for enhanced power
- Impaired resilience
- Risk for impaired resilience
- Readiness for enhanced resilience
- Chronic sorrow
- Stress overload
- Acute substance withdrawal syndrome
- Risk for acute substance withdrawal syndrome
- Autonomic dysreflexia
- Risk for autonomic dysreflexia
- neonatal abstinence syndrome
- Disorganized infant behavior
- Risk for disorganized infant behavior
- Readiness for enhanced organized infant behavior (Herdman, Kamitsuru, Lopes p. 393-394).
- Readiness for enhanced comfort
- Nausea
- Acute pain
- Chronic pain

- Chronic pain syndrome
- Labor pain
- Impaired comfort
- Readiness for enhanced comfort
  (Herdman, Kamitsuru, Lopes p. 549).
- Unilateral neglect
- Awareness of time, place, and person
- Acute confusion
- Risk for acute confusion
- Chronic confusion
- Labile emotional control
- Ineffective impulse control
- Deficient knowledge
- Readiness for enhanced knowledge
- Impaired memory
- Disturbed thought process
- Readiness for enhanced communication
- Impaired verbal communication
  (Herdman, Kamitsuru, Lopes p. 323-324).
- Sexual dysfunction
- Ineffective sexuality pattern
- Ineffective childbearing process
- Risk for ineffective childbearing process
- Readiness for enhanced childbearing process
- Risk for disturbed maternal-fetal dyad
  (Herdman, Kamitsuru, Lopes p.385).
- Delayed child development
- Risk for delayed child development
- Delayed infant motor development
- Risk for delayed infant motor development
  (Herdman, Kamitsuru, Lopes p.567).

Psychological Needs

Belongness & Love Needs

This psychological category deals with feelings of belonging, interpersonal relationships, intimacy, trust, acceptance, receiving and giving affection and love as well as being part of a group (family, friends, work, or special interests). The corresponding NANDA-I Nursing Domains® is Role Relationships.

- Impaired parenting
- Risk for impaired parenting
- Readiness for enhanced parenting
- Caregiver role strain
- Risk for caregiver role strain
- Risk for impaired attachment
- Disturbed family identity syndrome
- Risk for disturbed family identity syndrome
- Dysfunctional family processes
- Interrupted family processes
- Readiness for enhanced family processes
- Ineffective relationship
- Risk for ineffective relationship
- Readiness for enhanced relationship
- Parental role conflict
- Ineffective role performance
- Impaired social interaction (Herdman, Kamitsuru, Lopes p. 357-358).

Esteem Needs

Esteem needs pertain to individual self-esteem, dignity, achievement, mastery, independence and the desire for respect and reputation including status and prestige. The corresponding NANDA-I Nursing Domains® is Self-Perception.

- Hopelessness
- Readiness for enhanced hope
- Risk for compromised human dignity
- Disturbed personal identity
- Risk for disturbed personal identity
- Readiness for enhanced self-concept
- Chronic low Self-esteem
- Risk for chronic low self-esteem
- Situational low self-esteem
- Risk for situational low self-esteem
- Disturbed body image

(Herdman, Kamitsuru, Lopes p. 339-340)

Self-Fulfillment Needs

Self-Actualization

Self-Actualization pertains to the recognition and reaching of one's full potential, self-fullment, seeking personal growth, peak performance, and creative ideas. The corresponding NANDA-I Nursing Domains® are Health Promotion and Life Principles.

- Decreased diversional activity engagement
- Readiness for enhanced health literacy
- Sedentary lifestyle
- Risk for elopement attempt
- Frail elderly syndrome
- Risk for frail elderly syndrome
- Readiness for enhanced exercise engagement
- Deficient community health
- Risk-prone health behavior
- Ineffective health maintenance behaviors
- Ineffective health self-management
- Readiness for enhanced health self-management
- Ineffective family health self-management
- Ineffective home maintenance behaviors
- Risk for ineffective home maintenance behaviors
- Readiness for enhanced home maintenance behaviors
- Ineffective protection
  (Herdman, Kamitsuru, Lopes p. 187).
- Readiness for enhanced spiritual well-being
- Readiness for enhanced decision-making
- Decisional conflict
- Impaired emancipated decision-making
- Risk for impaired emancipated decision-making
- Readiness for enhanced emancipated decision-making
- Moral distress
- Impaired religiosity
- Risk for impaired religiosity
- Readiness for enhanced religiosity
- Spiritual distress
- Risk for spiritual distress

(Herdman, Kamitsuru, Lopes p. 447-448).

From Priorities to Test Plan

Nursing's aim is to provide client specific, preventative and holistic, care across the lifespan with respect to the cultural and spiritual needs of those we serve. Our ability to assess and initiate plans of care using the nursing process is the essence of our practice and should be based in both science and art. While the nursing process is a client centered problem solving method, the new language of the clinical judgment model is focused on the thought process and problem solving steps nurses utilize while implementing the nursing process. For this reason, I think it is important to overlay Maslow's Hierarchy of Needs with the NCLEX-RN® Test Plan. As a reminder, the most accurate test plan information is obtained from the current NCSBN NCLEX-RN® Test Plan website. Here is a link to the current Next Generation NCLEX, NCLEX-RN® Test Plan Effective April 2023.

The main reason I want to cross reference these items is to show you how important care plans are to NCLEX-RN® and practice success. We have already established that Maslow's Hierarchy of Needs is integrated in the Nursing Process. If you compare the approximate number of weighted questions in each client needs categories of NCLEX-RN®, to the percentage of NANDA-I® nursing diagnoses categorized by Maslow's Hierarchy of Needs the numbers are very proportionally similar.

NCLEX-RN®Test Plan Client Needs Categories, Competencies and Sample Content Cross-Referenced with Maslow's Hierarchy of Needs

NCLEX-RN®Client Needs / Percentage Questions	**Maslow's Hierarchy of Needs Category / Total Number NANDA-I Nursing Diagnoses**
Safe and Effective Care Environment: Management of Care ~ 15-21%	
Safe and Effective Care Environment: Safety and Infection Control ~ 10-16%	
Health Promotion and Maintenance ~ 6-12%	Self-Fulfillment Needs = 11.2%
Psychosocial Integrity ~ 6-12%	Psychological Needs = 8.81%
Physiological Integrity: Basic Care and Comfort ~ 6-12%	Basic Needs = 79.91 %
Physiological Integrity: Pharmacological and Parenteral Therapies ~ 13-19%	
Physiological Integrity: Reduction of Risk Potential ~ 9-15%	
Physiological Integrity ~ Physiological Adaptation ~ 11-17%	

Now let's break down each of the NCLEX-RN® Client Needs areas by competencies, sample content, and Maslow's corresponding Needs. You will need to go back to the previous sections to review the specific nursing diagnoses under each category of Maslow's Hierarchy of Needs. For consistency and familiarity, I will keep the Client Needs listed in the same order as the NCLEX-RN® test plan. I have bulleted the sample content so you can use it as a to-do list for your concepts you need to review. The following competencies and sample items are taken directly from the NCLEX-RN® April 2023 test plan and have not been paraphrased. ***Remember this book is a supplement and should never take the place of using the original NCLEX-RN test plan.***

Safe & Effective Care Environment: Safety & Infection Control

Corresponding Maslow's Hierarchy of Needs

Safety Needs

NCLEX-RN® Competencies

- Assess client for allergies and intervene as needed
- Assess client care environment
- Promote staff safety
- Protect client from injury
- Properly identify client when providing care
- Verify appropriateness and accuracy of a treatment order
- Participate in emergency planning and response
- Use ergonomic principles when providing care
- Following procedures for handling biohazardous and hazardous materials Educate client on safety issues
- Acknowledge and document practice errors and near misses
- Report, intervene, and/or escalate unsafe practice of health care personnel (e.g. substance abuse, improper care, staffing practices)
- Facilitate appropriate and safe use of equipment
- Follow security plan and procedures (e.g. newborn security, violence, controlled access)
- Apply principles of infection prevention (e.f. hand hygiene, aseptic technique, isolation, sterile technique, universal/standard enhanced barrier precautions) Educate client and staff regarding infection prevention measures Follow requirements when using restraints.

NCLEX-RN®Sample Content

- Accident/Error/Injury Prevention
- Emergency Response Plan
- Ergonomic Principles
- Handling Hazardous and Infectious Materials
- Home Safety
- Reporting of Incident/Event/Irregular Occurrence/Variance
- Safe Use of Equipment
- Security Plan
- Standard Precautions/Transmission-Based Precautions/Surgical Asepsis Use of Restraints/Safety Devices

Health Promotion & Maintenance

Corresponding Maslow's Hierarchy of Needs

Belongingness & Love Needs, Esteem Needs, Self-Actualization, & Physiological Needs

NCLEX-RN® Competencies

- Provide care and education for the newborn, infant, and toddler client from birth through 2 years
- Provide care and education for the preschool, school age and adolescent client ages 3 through 17 years
- Provide care and education for the adult client ages 18 through 64
- Provide care and education for the adult client ages 65 and older
- Provide prenatal care and education
- Provide care and education to an antepartum client or a client in labor
- Provide postpartum care and education
- Assess and educate clients about health risks based on family, population, and community
- Plan and/or participate in community health education
- Educate client about preventative care and health maintenance recommendations
- Provide resources to minimize communication barriers
- Perform targeted screening assessments (e.g. vision, nutrition, depression)
- Educate client about prevention and treatment of high risk health behaviors
- Assess client ability to manage care in home environment and plan care accordingly
  Perform comprehensive health assessment

NCLEX-RN® Sample Content

- Aging Process
- Ante-/Intra-/Postpartum and Newborn Care
- Developmental Stages and Transitions
- Health Promotion / Disease Prevention
- Health Screening
- High-Risk Behaviors
- Lifestyle Choices
- Self-Care
- Techniques of Physical Assessment

Psychosocial Integrity

Corresponding Maslow's Hierarchy of Needs

Physiological Needs, Safety Needs, Belongingness & Love Needs, Esteem Needs, & Self-Actualization

NCLEX-RN® Competencies

- Assess client for abuse or neglect and report, intervene, and/or escalate
- Incorporate behavioral management techniques when caring for a client
- Assess client for substance abuse and/or toxicities and intervene as appropriate (e.g. dependency, withdrawal)
- Assess client's ability to cope with life changes and provide support
- Assess the potential for violence and use safety precautions
- Incorporate client cultural practices and beliefs when planning and providing care
- Provide end-of-life care and education to clients
- Assess client support system to aid in plan of care
- Provide care for a client experiencing grief or loss
- Provide care and education for acute and chronic psychosocial health issues (e.g. addictions/dependencies, depression, dementia, eating disorders) Assess psychosocial factors influencing care and plan interventions (e.g.
- occupational, spiritual, environmental, financial)
- Provide appropriate care for a client experiencing visual, auditory, and/or cognitive alterations
- Recognize non-verbal cues to physical and/or psychological stressors
- Use therapeutic communication techniques
- Promote a therapeutic environment

NCLEX-RN® Sample Content

- Abuse or Neglect
- Behavioral Interventions
- Chemical and Other Dependencies/Substance Use Disorder
- Coping Mechanisms
- Crisis Intervention
- Cultural Awareness/Cultural Influences on Health
- End-of-Life Care

- Family Dynamics
- Grief and Loss
- Mental Health Concepts
- Religious and Spiritual Influences on Health
- Sensory/Perceptual Alterations
- Stress Management
- Support Systems
- Therapeutic Communication and Environment

Physiological Integrity: Basic Comfort & Care

Corresponding Maslow's Hierarchy of Needs

Physiological Needs, & Safety Needs

NCLEX-RN® Competencies

- Assist client to compensate for physical or sensory impairment (e.g. assistive devices, positioning)
- Assess and manage client with an alteration in bowel and bladder elimination
- Perform irrigations (e.g. of bladder, ear, eye)
- Perform skin assessment and implement measures to maintain skin integrity
- Apply, maintain, or remove orthopedic devices
- Implement measures to promote circulation (e.g. active or passive range of motion, positioning and mobilization)
- Assess client for pain and intervene as appropriate
- Recognize complementary therapies and identify potential benefits and contraindications (e.g. aromatherapy, acupressure, supplements) Provide non-pharmacological comfort measures
- Elevate the client's nutritional status and intervene as needed
- Provide client nutrition through tube feedings
- Evaluate client intake and output and intervene as needed
- Assess client performance of activities of daily living and assist when needed
- Perform post-mortem care
- Assess client sleep/rest pattern and intervene as needed

NCLEX-RN®Sample Content

- Assistive Devices
- Elimination
- Mobility/Immobility
- Non-Pharmacological Comfort Interventions
- Nutrition and Oral Hydration
- Personal Hygiene
- Rest and Sleep

Physiological Integrity: Pharmacological & Parenteral Therapies

Corresponding Maslow's Hierarchy of Needs

Safety Needs

NCLEX-RN® Competencies

- Administer blood products and evaluate client response
- Access and/or maintain central venous access devices
- Perform calculation needed for medication administration
- Evaluate client response to medication
- Prepare and administer medications using rights of medication administration Review pertinent data prior to medication administration (e.g. contraindications, lab results, allergies, potential interactions)
- Participate in medication reconciliation process
- Titrate dosage of medication based on assessment and ordered parameters
- Dispose of medications safely
- Handle and maintain medication in a safe and controlled environment
- Evaluate appropriateness and accuracy of medication order for client
- Handle and administer high-risk medications safely
- Monitor intravenous infusion and maintain site
- Administer medications for pain management
- Handle and administer controlled substances within regulatory guidelines
- Administer parenteral nutrition and evaluate client response

NCLEX-RN® Sample Content

- Adverse Effects/Contraindications/Side Effects/Interactions
- Blood and Blood Products
- Central Venous Access Devices
- Dosage Calculations
- Expected Actions/Outcomes
- Medication Administration
- Parenteral/Intravenous Therapies
- Pharmacological Pain Management
- Total Parenteral Nutrition

Physiological Integrity: Reduction of Risk Potential

Corresponding Maslow's Hierarchy of Needs

Physiological Needs, & Safety Needs

NCLEX-RN® Competencies

- Assess and respond to changes and trends in client vital signs
- Perform testing within scope of practice (e.g. electrocardiogram, glucose monitoring)
- Monitor the results of diagnostic testing and intervene as needed
- Obtain blood specimens\
- Obtain specimens other than blood for diagnostic testing
- Insert, maintain, or remove a nasal/oral gastrointestinal tube
- Insert, maintain or remove a urinary catheter
- Insert, maintain, or remove a peripheral intravenous line
- Maintain percutaneous feeding tube
- Apply and/or maintain devices used to promote venous return (e.g. anti-embolic stocking, sequential compression devices)
- Use precautions to prevent injury and/or complications associated with a procedure or diagnosis
- Evaluate client responses to procedures and treatment
- Recognize trends and changes in client condition and intervene as needed
- Perform focused assessments
- Educate client about treatments and procedures
- Provide preoperative care
- Manage client during a procedure with moderate sedation
- Manage client following a procedure with moderate sedation

NCLEX-RN®Sample Content

- Changes/Abnormalities in Vital Signs
- Diagnostic Tests
- Laboratory Values
- Potential for Alterations in Body Systems
- Potential for Complications of Diagnostic Tests/Treatment/Procedures
- Potential for Complications from Surgical Procedures and Health Alterations
- System-Specific Assessments
- Therapeutic Procedures

Physiological Integrity: Physiological Adaptation

Corresponding Maslow's Hierarchy of Needs

Physiological Needs, & Safety Needs

NCLEX-RN® Competencies

- Assist with invasive procedures (e.g. central line, thoracentesis, bronchoscopy)
- Implement and monitor phototherapy
- Maintain optimal temperature of client
- Monitor and care for clients on a ventilator
- Monitor and maintain devices and equipment used for drainage (e.g. surgical wound drains, chest tube suction, negative pressure wound therapy)
- Perform and manage care of client receiving peritoneal dialysis
- Perform suctioning
- Perform wound care and dressing change
- Provide ostomy care and education (e.g. tracheal, enteral)
- Provide pulmonary hygiene (e.g. chest physiotherapy, incentive spirometry)
- Provide postoperative care

NCLEX-RN® Competencies(cont.)

- Manage the care of the client with a fluid and electrolyte imbalance
- Monitor and maintain arterial lines
- Manage the care of a client with a pacing device
- Manage the care of a client on telemetry
- Manage the care of a client receiving hemodialysis or continuous renal replacement therapy
- Manage the care of a client with alteration in hemodynamics, tissue perfusion, and hemostasis
- Educate client regarding an acute or chronic condition
- Manage the care of a client with impaired ventilation/oxygenation
- Evaluate the effectiveness of the treatment plan for a client with an acute or chronic diagnosis
- Perform emergency care procedures
- Identify pathophysiology related to an acute or chronic condition
- Recognize sign and symptoms of client complications and intervene

NCLEX-RN® Sample Content

- Alterations in Body Systems
- Fluid and Electrolyte Imbalances
- Hemodynamics
- Illness Management
- Medical Emergencies
- Pathophysiology
- Unexpected Response to Therapies
  (NCSBN, Effective Date April 2023)

HOW to Study

This information originated nine years ago to help me make sure that I was giving consistent information to every student. It was during individual sessions I realized how extremely overwhelmed students are by current course work, thoughts of graduation, life decisions, and the licensure exam. They are either too anxious to do anything, or they try so many different things that nothing seems to work. It wasn't long before this information developed into a document that I share with each of my students. In addition to listening and helping them create a personalized study plan, I want them to feel confident they now have an organized process of preparing for NCLEX-RN®. This section will review essential resources, provide suggestions on time management and suggest a systematic way to study. I admit, this is an intense to-do list. Not everything on this list can or should be done during the last semester of school. These are all the things I recommend you do before you schedule your exam. Just like a good care plan book I have listed things by prioritized goals, then the corresponding tasks.

GATHER WHAT YOU NEED

The goal of these tasks is to have everything you need easily accessible. You want to have things organized so that when it is time to study there won't be any excuses to procrastinate. It is best if you have a dedicated location to study and can leave everything out. Getting organized will also build confidence knowing that you have everything you need to be successful.

Create a NCLEX-RN® Study Binder

- Print and read the applicable NCSBN NCLEX-RN® Test Plan
- Print and read the current NCSBN NCLEX-RN® Candidate Bulletin. Knowing all about the process of applying and what to expect will ease many of your anxieties.
- **Add note paper and dividers.** You may find it easiest to organize by concept, body systems, Maslow's Hierarchy of Needs®, or NCLEX-RN® Client Needs categories. If you are using a NCLEX-RN® content review product, online or in-person, you might consider organizing your notes in a similar order.
- **Add a legal pad to keep a To-Do list going.** I generally recommend that you use this for concepts you need to look at in greater depth. It's also good to list questions you need to look up later. This list will be constantly changing. Your To-Do list may spawn its own to-do list and you will likely need a Do-Not list. Remember to put these items in your study planner or daily calendar.
- **Include your study planner**. We will discuss time management in the coming sections.

- **Get your computer, textbooks, reference books, class notes, index cards, recorded lectures or any other study aids you used**. **Be sure to include this book so you have the list of nursing diagnoses organized by Maslow's Hierarchy of Needs®.** You will also need your favorite care plan book, a NCLEX-RN® review book of your choice, Med-Surg, Peds, OB, Psych, Fundamentals, Pharm books, drug, lab and procedures guides. Remember online programs you use. Make sure your username and password are written down so you don't waste time trying to get logged in. You want everything at your fingertips so you aren't disrupted having to stop and go get what you forgot.
- **Include any exit exam reports or predictive exam feedback.** If you need help understanding the report, ask your nursing faculty. Most predictive exams will be broken down by NCLEX-RN® client needs and or nursing concepts. Most products will generate remediation packets that include concepts you need to review based on the questions you missed.
- **Dedicate space to study and simulate as much of the testing environment as possible**. Conditioning is key to reducing test anxiety. The candidate bulletin will provide information about what to expect but don't hesitate calling the actual testing center you plan to use, if you have additional questions. I have found them to be very helpful with information, like room temperature or if additional fans may be running, etc.
- **STOP BAD HABITS NOW.** You won't be able to listen to music during the exam, so don't do it while you study.

ASSESS

The goal of these tasks is to figure out exactly where to begin. You will not have to relearn everything that has been covered in nursing school. Right now you are reinforcing the most important things you learned. At the end of every task, add things you don't remember to the big To-Do list. The tasks listed below are in no particular order.

- **Figure out what you know and know what you don't know.** This really is one of the most important things you can do to prepare. Most students have no idea where to begin. As always, it's best to start where you are. I know it's scary but you will likely be pleasantly surprised at the amount of things you won't need to relearn.
- ***Know how your electronic resources work and maximize their potential.*** For example, an online/phone app may be designed as a full content review, a conditioning tool, or both. When reviewing products consider the following. Does the product accommodate your particular learning style? Does the product gather accumulative information with detailed feedback? Are their predictive exams and are they comprehensive or adaptive? Do their practice exams look and navigate like NCLEX-RN®? How reliable is their product? Do they publish a success rate? Do they offer a money back guarantee? How large is their question bank? I also recommend maximizing the resource of one product before moving to the next. Working on multiple platforms at the same time can be very confusing and not a productive use of time.
- ***Find out what resources are available on your campus.*** Most offer counseling services for test taking anxiety. Some of these services may be free as a student but may not be accessible after graduation. On a side note, if you currently use testing accommodations, contact your board of nursing to see what that process would be for NCLEX-RN ®. There may be additional documentation and paperwork for this process.
- ***Review the test plan paying close attention to client needs categories, competencies and sample items.*** This will help you stay focused on what is most important to study now.
- ***Review the nursing diagnoses prioritized by Maslow's Hierarchy of Needs.*** Just the diagnoses. You will come back and study specific care plans and nursing interventions later. Remember right now you are just assessing.
- ***Review the Head-to-Toe Integrated physical exam.*** A great way to study this is to hand write it as if you were charting a normal exam. Leave blanks where you can't remember. Then, look up what's normal and fill in the blanks. I suggest this weekly until you take your licensure exam.

- ***Review the Stages of Pregnancy, Fetal Development including circulation.***
- ***Review all stages of Growth and Development, birth to death.***
- ***Go over routine immunization schedules for children and adults. Not the catch-up schedule.***

- ***Stages of Death and Dying.***
- ***Implications of Lab Values.***
- ***Cultural Awareness.***
- ***Common prefixes and suffixes.***
- ***Principles of teaching and learning.***
- ***Crisis Intervention.***
- ***Care of the Moderately Sedated.***
- ***Drug Classifications.***
- ***Dimensional Analysis.***
- ***Speciality diets and nutritional value of foods.***
- ***Delegation.***
- ***Scope of Practice.***
- ***Commonalities of Nurse Practice Acts and Legal aspects.***
- ***Pathophysiology. Remember two thirds of the exam will be safety and physiological needs. This is another great reason to study care plans in these categories.***

Again, at this point you are assessing to determine how to budget your time. Some things will have to and should wait. Organize the To-Do list. Look for patterns and be logical about how you can add these things to your already busy schedule.

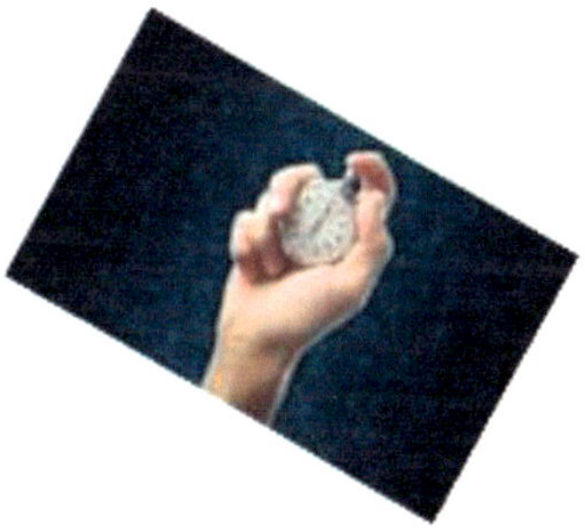

My Best Advice is to Catch Up Quickly

- Know the integrated physical head-to-toe.
- Relearn stages of growth and development.

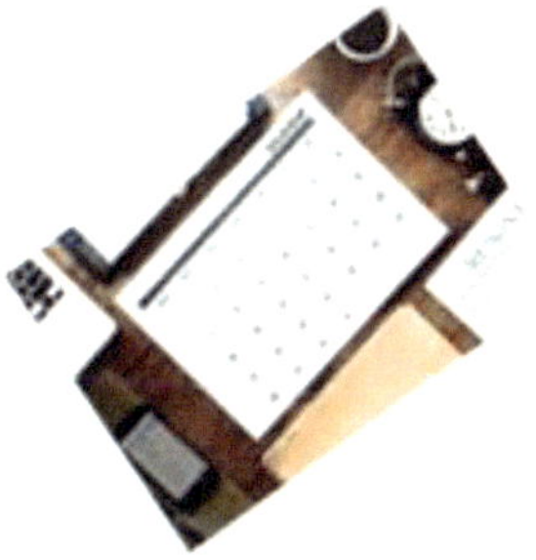

- STUDY CARE PLANS organized by Maslow's Hierarchy of Needs!
- Do a small batch of hard practice questions (10-20) after every concept studied.

Time Management

Good time management allows you to properly prepare you for the licensure exam, reduces anxiety and strengthens confidence. Most of all, efficient time management with frequent assessments and readjustments will help you reach your goals faster than just waiting to see what happens. The following are just a few pointers, in no particular order.

- ***Find a study/personal planner that is aesthetically pleasing.*** Either hard copy or online is fine. Choose whatever format you are most likely to use. It should have some room for additional tasks or a place to write down what you need to prioritize. Color Coding works well too.
- ***Fill in the essential commitments first.*** Remember Maslow's Hierarchy of Needs applies to you too. Start with a sleep/wake schedule. Allow plenty of time to shower, dress, shop for essentials, prepare and eat your meals, put gas in your car, commute to school and or work, get to and from class and clinical, travel home to see family. Then continue with school assignments and clinical schedules. You will plug in NCLEX-RN® study time after that. Set aside time for both content review and practice questions in the beginning. You will progress to nothing but practice questions later.
- ***Be realistic!*** Make a schedule that you would want to have. Include things you enjoy, time with friends or other social obligations you find fulfilling. You can always cut back on those activities if you find you are not able to get the needed things done.
- ***Make your bed and tidy your living space before you leave each day.*** You may wonder if I'm writing this to see if you are paying attention. I'm not. It's really important! Clutter increases stress. Completing small daily tasks builds positive self-esteem and a sense of achievement. If all else fails and your day has been worse than bad, you will at least come home to one accomplishment and a clean space. If you still feel defeated, remember tomorrow is another opportunity to try again.
- ***Look for gaps in time and multi-task.*** If you are commuting, cleaning or doing laundry, listen to podcasts, audio lessons or recorded notes.
- ***Overlay your current course work with your content review.*** This is really important. For example, if you are covering neurological care in class and neuro. is on your list of content to review, put that on your schedule for now and not two weeks after your unit exam.

- ***Ask for help or delegate what you can't get done.*** You may not have any financial assistance and have to work for the bare necessities. If that is the case then talk with your faculty. There may be resources on campus to help with non-traditional expenses. Take a look at your budget. If you need more time to study and TV is a distraction you might consider changing your cable plan. Talk with your parents or employer to see if working less outside of school is an option, at least until you pass your licensure exam. Chances are good that effective time management will decrease your stress and improve your relationships with others. It will definitely make you feel better about yourself.
- ***Do what you dread most first.*** This will motivate you to do more and stay on task.
- ***Add layers of accountability.*** Tell your family and friends about your plans. If they are aware of the extra time you will be studying they will be less likely to tempt you with activities you didn't make time for. Put your schedule on the refrigerator, sticky notes on your bathroom mirror, encouraging notes in your car or set alerts on your phone to keep you on task. Turn off countdown trackers if they are causing you anxiety.
- ***Avoid Distractions.*** Set your phone to silent so alerts, calls, and texts go to an automatic response.
- ***Remember your why!*** What or who made you want to become a nurse? Think of all the family, friends, classmates, and faculty that have helped along the way. You are so close to reaching this goal and I promise your hard work will pay off. This will motivate you and help you find the most important priorities.

When you Study

This section is dedicated to general reminders to help you find a systematic way to study. Again, you want NCLEX-RN® preparation to be efficient and effective. It is very important to know your learning style and what type of studying works best for you. By no means am I suggesting that you start doing everything differently. You have obviously been very successful or you won't have made it to this point. I want you to do what works best for you. You need to maximize your strengths and minimize your weaknesses. Tasks listed below are in no particular order.

- ***LET STUDY BE STUDY AND PRACTICE QUESTIONS BE CONDITIONING.*** What I am referring to here is avoid doing practice questions in study mode. Practice questions should simulate high-steaks NCLEX-RN® testing. Anytime you are answering practice questions incorrectly, stop!, figure out what content you are missing, then go back and review it again. Missing a lot of questions because you don't know the content is a huge waste of time. It also starts a very negative feedback loop of self-defeating language.
- ***Study content, review the corresponding care plans, goals and interventions, then do a set number of hard practice questions on that exact same content.*** If you feel you are veering off track when studying, re-visit the test plan. You can also go over content from a NCLEX-RN® review book. If you feel you are studying too in-depth, look back over the care plans then stop and try some more practice questions.
- ***Content, Care Plans, then Practice Questions.*** Yes. I meant to say that again. It is that important.
- ***Take handwritten notes***. It really will help you remember better than typing.
- ***Do practice questions in test mode. Review your results, reading all rationales for wrong and right answers.*** Add content to your To-Do list as needed.
- ***When you feel confident you understand the content material, switch to nothing but hard practice questions.*** You can always add more content reviews to your To-Do list if you run across something you need to review.
- ***Dedicate a minimum of two hours a day for nothing but hard practice questions.*** Remember conditioning is key! Your goal is to get an eighty five question exam.
- ***Do at least one practice session of hard questions for a minimum of four to five hours***. If you start getting more than eighty five questions or go past two hours, you will at least know that you can sit there and maintain your concentration for the maximum amount of time.
- ***Consider recording a practice session.*** You will be recorded during your licensure exam and it might help ease some testing anxiety. You can also see if you have any test taking habits that could be viewed as suspicious behavior.
- ***Consider a private tutor***, especially if you don't feel you are getting what you need during school. You should ask for extra help as needed.
- ***Take an in-person NCLEX-RN® review course***. If your school does not have one as part of your curriculum, find one. This is definitely one thing that is worth the added expense.

Some companies offer a money back guarantee, or your new employer may reimburse you, so ask and shop around.

I did not cover specific review products for several reasons. Not every product meets every student's needs. Products change quickly, be it substance, services, price, availability. I don't want to interject bias based on products I use or products I may be familiar with. I do not feel comfortable recommending products I am unfamiliar with or recommend specific resources based on informal student feedback. I have never been paid or received incentive to endorse any product. I have also chosen not to cover test taking techniques. I don't consider myself an authority in this area. There are many resources available online, in books or during a designated review course to help you with test taking techniques. Again, a large volume of practice questions is essential to your success.

When to Schedule the Exam

Most students want to know when they should take NCLEX®. I recommend having completed a minimum of three thousand hard practice questions with good success and at least two or three positive predictor tests saying you are ready to take the exam. Different preparation products have different suggestions. Feeling confident in your process and preparation is essential. If ever there was an exam to over prepare for, it is this one. Plus, you want to condition yourself for an eighty five question, two hour exam and not the one hundred and fifty question, five hour exam. ***I can tell you with one hundred percent certainty****, you will pass this exam on your first attempt if you make sure you are ready before you take it.* Remember, you are the one scheduling the exam. It's not pre scheduled for you.

Narrowing Your Practice Gap

The practice gap is not a new term and is certainly nothing you aren't already familiar with. How many times in clinical practice have you heard, "this is not the book answer"? What you see in practice and what you see on exams are sometimes different. That doesn't mean that the NCLEX-RN® does not represent today's nursing practice. NCSBN® goes to great lengths to make sure that it does. The practice gap I am talking about is how long it takes you to transition from a student who can pass a licensure exam that measures a minimum amount of safety, into the role of an entry-level nurse that functions competently in today's workforce. It's one of the reasons we have the current NCLEX-RN® test plan.

I want your time as an entry level nurse to be meaningful and inspiring. You will be very task oriented for the first few years. You won't have the experiences from hundreds of clients to fall back on and you probably won't have time to leave the bedside to go look many things up. You have to rely on your assessment skills, pay close attention to minute changes, then be brave enough to initiate those often very simple, nursing interventions from a standardized care plan book. If it doesn't work, you just keep trying. The good news is, most of the time the interventions do work but you have to know them.

So, what if you start today? Become more familiar with the most basic nursing diagnoses. Rely on Maslow's Hierarchy of Needs®. Learn how to set appropriate goals and know what interventions aim toward those goals. It will give you the confidence you need to put a plan in action. You will feel more confident and your patients feel safer, knowing you are their nurse.

Conclusion

I hope I have communicated well how much I care about your success as a student and a nurse. I wish you the best of luck in life and on your nursing journey. Most of all I sincerely appreciate the time you spent using this book. I hope that you will study and standardized care plans well into your nursing practice. The tasks suggested in this book are not adding more things to your list of things to do. It is reorganizing what you should already be doing so that you can be efficient and effective in your preparation and the care you provide.

Ultimately, the decision to do more is all up to you. Since you've read this far, chances are good that you are better than most. You care a lot, study extra and work even harder. No one has ever said nursing is easy but it is definitely worth it! I'll finish with what I always tell my students and new nurses.

"No one said the nudge out of this nest is gentle, but it is done with great love."

Blessings for a long and happy Nursing career!

Sincerely,

Lori A. Ballard MSN, RN

For additional questions, comments, or to request a consult, please email
keystosuccesslballard@gmail.com

Special Thanks

I would like to thank my husband, Brent. You are the love of life and my greatest support. To my parents, children, grandchildren, friends, and colleagues. I love you and appreciate all the encouragement you freely give. Nursing has been very kind to me. I am fortunate to have had wonderful mentors and co-workers throughout my career. I have cared for so many patients who will never know how our experiences together touched my very soul. I am thankful for each and every one of you. I wish you all Peace and Blessings beyond measure.

Works Cited

Armstrong, Nancy, et al. "Mentoring Program for Graduating Bachelor of Science in Nursing Students." *Kentucky Journal of Excellence in College Teaching and Learning*, vol. 15, 2018, pp. 11-17.

Doenges, Marilynn E., et al. *Nurse's Pocket Guide: Diagnoses, Prioritized Interventions, and Rationales*. F. A. Davis Company, 2022.

Hawkins, Joellen W. *The Historical Evolution of Theories and Conceptual Models for Nursing*. Historical Materials (060). 1987, https://files.eric.ed.gov/fulltext/ED284969.pdf. Accessed 3 January 2024.

Haws, Jon, and step guide. "5 Tips on How to Master NCLEX Test Questions." *NURSING.com blog*, https://blog.nursing.com/master-nursing-questions. Accessed 3 January 2024.

Herdman, T. Heather, et al. *NANDA International, Inc. Nursing Diagnoses 2020-2023 Definitions and Classifications*. Twelfth ed., New York, Stuttgart, Delhi, Rio de Janeiro, Thieme, 2019.

Herdman, T. Heather, and Camila Lopes. *Supplement to NANDA International Nursing Diagnoses: Definitions and Classification 2021-2023 (12th Edition)*. Edited by T. Heather Herdman and Camila Lopes, Thieme Medical Publishers, 2023. m, jose.
"✍." *YouTube*, 30 August 2022,
https://www.google.com/search?q=history+of+nanda+international&rlz=1C1GCEA_enUS982US982&oq=history+o&gs_lcrp=EgZjaHJvbWUqCAgAEEUYJxg7MggIABBFGCcYOzIOCAEQRRgnGDsYgAQYigUyBggCEEUYOzIGCAMQRRhAMgYIBBBFGDkyCggFEAAYsQMYgAQyBggGEEUYPDIGCAcQRRg80gEIMzQ0M2owajSoAgC. Accessed 3 January 2024.

Mary, Dellefield E. "Interdisciplinary Care Planning and the Witten Care Plan in Nursing Homes: A Critical Review." *The Gerontologist*, vol. 46, no. 1, 2006, pp. 128-133. https://doi.org/10.1093/geront/46.1.128. Accessed Google December 2023.
Maslow, Abraham H. "A Theory of Human Motivation." *Psychological Review*, vol. 50, no. 4, 1943, pp. 1-27, https://www.academia.edu/9415670/A_Theory_of_Human_Motivation_Abraham_H_Maslow_Psychological_Review_Vol_50_No_4_July_1943. Accessed 18 December 2023.
"NANDA_NursingDiagnoses_21-23_Sample." *Thieme Medical Publishers*, https://web.thieme.com/images/stories/epaper-NANDA_NursingDiagnoses_21/#0. Accessed 3 January 2024.

"Nursing orders Definition." *Law Insider*, https://www.lawinsider.com/dictionary/nursing-orders. Accessed 3 January 2024. Orlando, I.J. "The dynamic nurse-patient relationship." 1961, NewYork: Putnam's.

Simmons, Lydia. "Download Abstract Triangle Free Transparent Image HQ HQ PNG

Image." *FreePNGImg*, 28 July 2023, https://freepngimg.com/png/172022-abstract-triangle-free-transparent-image-hq. Accessed 3 January 2024.

"2023 NCLEX-RN® Test Plan." *NCSBN*, https://www.nclex.com/files/2023_RN_Test%20Plan_English_FINAL.pdf. Accessed 3 January 2024.

Image. "American Photographic Artists", 2 Feb 2024, https://www.google.com/search?sca_esv=d07f85f75a168a72&rlz=1C1GCEA_enUS982US982&sxsrf=ACQVn09Q9pPqGnMvraBNy2WBjyNeqJbfHg:1706894329296&q=keys+to+success&uds=AMwkrPsq60QolqASVFXM5G2JGGO0ku40InRkLbGazbW5FuIv1B4H8n5-Rlcr_2GcBucTiP5vqWpyHUK1_gP7M3F3Sjb5c1V0ddda5Fmw1hn89eaVG9pPD5gljcRIfDBvki6toyyAPNuI&udm=2&sa=X&ved=2ahUKEwj7tKrxlI2EAxVXv4kEHUHXB5QQtKgLegQIFhAB&biw=1536&bih=735&dpr=1.25#vhid=3Aus6auADLvW2M&vssid=mosaic

Image. "Maslow's Hierarchy of Needs", 5 Feb 2024, https://www.thoughtco.com/maslows-hierarchy-of-needs-45825

Made in the USA
Las Vegas, NV
08 November 2026

57690472R00026